Daniel Diet: 20 Minute Recipes

25 Delectable, Nutritious, & Fulfilling Meals in Just 20 Minutes

Disclaimer

What Will You Find in This Book

The Daniel Diet is a healthy lifestyle plan, which provides all of the essential nutrients your body needs, while ensuring that you achieve your objective of losing those extra pounds. It is a brilliant way to start living a healthy life by taking a biblical approach to life. This book contains some of the most delicious 20-minute recipes from the Daniel Diet, which are not only healthy but also so delicious that you cannot help but enjoy them.

The book has been created to provide all health enthusiasts a chance to whip up delicious and nutritious meals in just 20 minutes. Amaze your friends and family, by cooking for them, the recipes mentioned in this book. After reading this book, you will become an expert at 20-minute recipes.

So waste no more time on deliberating, start perusing through the book, and enjoy the culinary experience.

Contents

Daniel Diet 20 Minute Recipes

Nowadays, more and more people are moving their focus towards healthy lifestyle. Therefore, without wasting any time, let us start cooking some of the most delectable and scrumptious recipes out there.

Baked Broccoli Frittata

SERVES 3

Prep Time: 5 minutes   **Cooking Time:** 15 minutes

Nutritional Facts: Calories 132, Total Fat 3.6 g, Carbohydrates 2.8 g, Protein 19 g

Ingredients

6 large eggs

1 red onion, medium in size, finely chopped

1 tbsp parsley, finely chopped

1 clove of garlic, finely chopped

2 cups broccoli, coarsely chopped

3 tbsp Parmesan cheese

A healthy pinch of salt

1 tsp extra virgin olive oil

¼ tsp pepper

Directions

Place a non stick frying pan over medium high heat, add in the olive oil, and let it heat up. Add in the chopped onions, and cook until it starts to become soft and translucent. This will take 3 minutes. Add in the chopped parsley, garlic, and broccoli and cook, until the broccoli become bright green in color; this would again take 3-5 minutes. Make sure to stir continuously to prevent the ingredients from sticking to the pan. Season it with salt and pepper, taste and adjust the seasoning if required.

Take a mixing bowl, crack open the eggs in it and then whisk them until well beaten. Mix the broccoli mixture with the eggs, and then pour this mixture in a greased baking dish. Sprinkle the top of the mixture with parmesan cheese, make sure that it is spread out evenly, and then transfer the baking dish in a preheated oven, with its temperature set at 400°F. Let the mixture bake for 12-15 minutes, or until the frittata is firm and not wobbly in the centre. Take it out of the oven, use a sharp knife to make even portions, serve hot to your family, and enjoy!

Grilled Fish with Spicy Raw Salad

SERVES 3

Prep Time: 4 minutes   **Cooking Time:** 16 minutes

Nutritional Facts: Calories 180, Total Fat 2 g, Carbohydrates 23 g, Protein 16 g

Ingredients

The juice of 1 lime

1 lb halibut

1 tsp extra virgin olive oil

A healthy pinch of salt

2 cups purple or green cabbage, finely sliced

1 cup carrots, finely sliced then julienned

Ground Pepper, as required

2 tbsp organic almond butter

2 tsp rice wine vinegar

½ tsp cayenne pepper

Directions

Chop all of the ingredients as mentioned in the recipe and then set aside. Take a cooking brush, dip it in olive oil, and brush the halibut generously with it. Then place a grill over medium heat, and drizzle a tsp of olive oil in it. Once the grill is smoking hot, add the fish and let it cook on each side until the grill starts to become flaky. This will require 8 minutes on each side. While the fish is cooking, take a mixing bowl, add in the almond butter, then combine the rice wine vinegar, lime juice, carrots, cayenne pepper, and cabbage in it, and toss them around until all of the ingredients are thoroughly incorporated and the dressing is evenly spread out over the vegetables.

Once the fish is cooked, transfer it over a serving platter, and top it with the prepared vegetables. Serve and enjoy this delicious meal with your friends and family.

Ground Turkey

SERVES 3

Prep Time: 4 minutes   **Cooking T**

Nutritional Facts: Calories 250, Total Fat 1 g, Carbohy

Ingredients

10 cups water, for boiling

¾ lb ground turkey

2 cups gluten free pasta

1 head of broccoli

2 medium tomatoes, chopped

1 tsp yellow mustard

1 tbsp soy sauce, low sodium

½ cup chopped onion

1 tsp salt

1 tsp black pepper, freshly grinded

1 tsp extra virgin olive oil

Directions

Place a large saucepan over medium high heat, and add in the water in it. Bring it to boil. Add in the pasta in it and allow it to cook for 10 minutes or until it is soft and tender. While the pasta is cooking, place a large skillet over medium slow heat, drizzle a little bit of olive oil in it and place the ground turkey to cook. Cook the turkey until it starts getting golden brown in color; make sire to give it an occasional stir, so that the turkey does not stick to the pan.

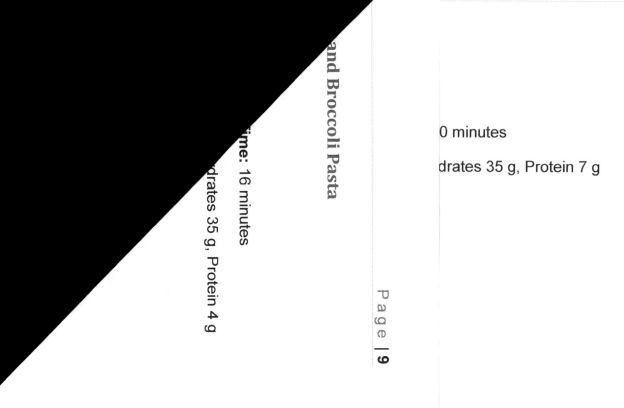

0 minutes

drates 35 g, Protein 7 g

and Broccoli Pasta

Time: 16 minutes

drates 35 g, Protein 4 g

Directions

Take a large bowl, add in the lettuce, onion, salsa, and avocado in it and then thoroughly mix it all together until all the ingredients are evenly combined, and coated with the mixture. Set the mixture aside for a couple of minutes, allowing the flavors to really come through. This will take about 5 minutes. Then take a tortilla, take half of the beans mixture, spread it over the tortilla evenly, and then top it vegetables. Wrap the tortilla in the style of a burrito, and then follow up with the remaining tortilla and vegetable mixture. Serve and enjoy this delicious and healthy burrito.

Balsamic Glazed Fish Fillets

SERVES 4

Prep Time: 10 minutes   **Cooking Time:** 10 minutes

Nutritional Facts: Calories 116, Total Fat 1 g, Carbohydrates 1.1 g, Protein 25 g

Ingredients

4 fish fillets, 6 oz each, skinless, ¾ to 1 inch in thickness

¼ cup balsamic vinegar

¼ cup extra virgin olive oil

4 lemon wedges

2 tsp shallots, finely chopped

2 tbsp each of chives, basil, thyme, and any other herb you like, finely chopped

1 tbsp parsley, finely chopped

2 cloves of garlic, medium in size, finely chopped

1 tsp oregano, finely chopped

½ tsp salt

½ tsp pepper, freshly grinded

Directions

Take a shallow dish, and put the fish in it, set aside. Take a mixing bowl, add in the vinegar, garlic, extra virgin olive oil, parsley, shallots, oregano, pepper and salt as required and then mix it all together until thoroughly combined. Pour this prepared mixture over the fish and then make sure that the fish is thoroughly coated with the mixture. Once done, allow it to marinade in a cold place for 5-8 minutes, as it will take only 2 minutes to prepare all of the ingredients. If you have, the time then set it aside to marinade in the refrigerator for at least 3-4 hours. Make sure that both sides of the fish are thoroughly covered with the mixture to allow the flavors to get soaked into the fish.

Then when you are ready, place a grill over medium high heat, and then drizzle a little bit of olive oil over it. When the grill starts to get smoking hot, place the fish on it and allow it to cook for 5 minutes on each side. The time can vary depending on the type of fish you have chosen to cook and its thickness. Grill it until it is cooked through and then transfer to a serving platter. Squeeze a little bit of lemon juice over it, topped with a few fresh herbs, and then serve and enjoy!

Cajun Roasted Cod

SERVES 1

Prep Time: 10 minutes   **Cooking Time:** 10 minutes

Nutritional Facts: Calories 110, Total Fat 1.5 g, Carbohydrates 1 g, Protein 16 g

Ingredients

3 oz saffron rice (optional)

1 piece ot cod, 4 oz

1 slice of onion

1 slices of tomatoes

2 tbsp canola oil

1 tsp Cajun spice mix

4 slices of bell pepper

½ oz herb oil (optional)

Directions

Take a baking sheet, grease with a little bit of canola oil, and then start adding layers of the slices vegetables. Take a small mixing bowl; add in the remaining tablespoon of olive oil, and whisk until the two are well combined. Add the spice mixture into the dish and rub the fish it on both sides, so that it is evenly spread. Place the cod over the vegetables, and then transfer the baking sheet in a preheated oven with its temperature set at 400°F. Let it bake for 10-12 minutes, until it is cooked through, then take it, transfer to a serving platter alo9ng with the vegetables, serve and enjoy!

Cast Iron Beef

SERVES 3

Prep Time: 3 minutes   **Cooking Time:** 17 minutes

Nutritional Facts: Calories 248, Total Fat 17 g, Carbohydrates 6 g, Protein 16 g

Ingredients

1 tsp Cajun spices

1 beef tenderloin, trimmed lean, cut into 4 pieces

1 oz canola oil

1 tsp all purpose seasoning

Directions

Combine all of the ingredients until the mixes are evenly incorporated with the beef, and then place it in a skillet with a little bit of canola oil in it. Sear all of the pieces on all sides in the skillet, for about a minute on each side, and then transfer the skillet in a preheated oven with its temperature set at 400°F. Allow it to bake for 10-12 minutes, then remove it from the oven and set aside for 4 minutes to rest. Transfer to a serving dish, serve, and enjoy with your friends and family.

Garden Cavatappi

SERVES 2

Prep Time: 5 minutes   **Cooking Time:** 15 minutes

Nutritional Facts: Calories 234, Total Fat 5 g, Carbohydrates 32 g, Protein 8 g

Ingredients

1 tbsp olive oil

1 tsp garlic, finely chopped

1 cup bell pepper, coarsely chopped

¼ cup Chinese egg plant, diced

½ cup zucchini, cubed

½ cup sweet onion, chopped into dices

½ Roma tomato, quartered

2 crimini mushrooms, quartered

½ oz shredded parmesan cheese

6 Kalamata olives, pitted and then sliced in half lengthwise.

2 cups cavatappi pasta

2 tbsp basil, fresh and finely chopped

1 cup marinara sauce

½ tsp all purpose seasoning

Directions

Boil the pasta as per the instructions given on its packet. Drain, drizzle with a little bit of water and set aside. This will take about 5 minutes. Then place a skillet over medium high heat, drizzle a little bit of olive oil in it, and then add in the garlic. Cook the garlic for a minute, then add in the zucchini, onions, eggplants, and peppers, and cook them until they start to become tender. This will take about 2-3 minutes. Add in the tomato, basil, and olives, and mix until well combined. Cook it for another 1 or 2 minutes, until the tomatoes start getting tender. Add in the sauce and combine it until well incorporated.

Pour in the pasta and combine until evenly incorporated and the pasta is completely mixed with the rest of the ingredients. Taste and adjust the seasoning if required, and then transfer to a serving bowl, and sprinkle the parmesan cheese and herbs. Serve and enjoy!

Whole Grain Granola

SERVES 16

Prep Time: 5 minutes   **Cooking Time:** 15 minutes

Nutritional Facts: Calories 150, Total Fat 5 g, Carbohydrates 19 g, Protein 7 g

Ingredients

2 cups regular rolled oats

1 ½ cups cashew nuts, chopped

1/8 tsp nutmeg powder

1-cup wheat cereal flakes

½ cup sunflower seeds, shelled

½ cup pumpkin seeds, shelled

½ cup coconut, shredded

¼ cup toasted wheat germ

¼ cup sesame seeds

1/4 cup cooking oil

1 ½ tsp vanilla extract

½-cup peanut butter

¾ tsp cinnamon powder

Directions

Take a roasting pan, grease it and then add in the oats, cashews, wheat cereal flakes, sunflower seeds, shredded coconut, pumpkin seeds, sesame seeds and wheat germ, and combine it until thoroughly incorporated. Add the remaining ingredients in another mixing bowl and combine until well incorporated. Drizzle the mixture from the bowl over the mixture in the roasting pan and then toss until well combined. Transfer the roasting pan in a preheated oven with its temperature set at 325oF and allow the mixture to cook for 15 minutes. It will be light brown in color by then. Make sure to give it a stir every 4-5 minutes. Take the granola out of the oven, and transfer it to a piece of foil and spread it out evenly. These can be stored for up to two weeks, in an airtight container. Serve, and enjoy!

**Prep T

Nutritional Facts:

Ingredients

2 tbsp extra virgin olive

½ tsp cayenne pepper

1 onion, medium in size

3 cups vegetable stock

1 can of black beans, d

2 cans of pumpkin pure

1 can of diced tomatoe

1 cup of soy milk

1 tbsp curry powder

1 ½ tsp cumin powder

Salt

20 chives, finely chopped

Directions

Place a large pot over medium heat, add in a little bit of oil in it and allow it to heat up. Once the oil is hot enough, add in the onions and sauté them for 5 minutes until translucent, then add in the stock. Stir and then add the tomatoes, pumpkin puree, black beans, and mix it until well combined. Lower the heat to medium low and allow the concoction to simmer, before adding in the curry, soy milk, cumin, salt and cayenne pepper. Taste and adjust the seasoning, if required and then allow it to simmer for 10 minutes, before pouring into a serving bowl, garnishing with chives, and serving. Enjoy!

Vegetable and B

S

Prep Time: 5 min

Nutritional Facts: Calorie

Ingredients

1 cup mixed vegetab

1 can tomato so

1 can white

Directi

C

...ean Soup

...ERVES 2

...utes   **Cooking Time:** 15 minutes

...s 50, Total Fat 1.5 g, Carbohydrates 9 g, Protein 2 g

...es, frozen

...up

...beans

...ons

...mbine all the ingredients in a pot. Place the pot over medium low heat, concoction to come to boil, and then reduce the heat to low. Allow it to simmer for 15-17 minutes until the vegetables start getting tender. Make sure to give it an occasional stir, to prevent it from sticking to the bottom of the pot. Pour into a serving bowl, serve hot and enjoy with your friends and family.

Savory Tofu Stew

SERVES 16

Prep Time: 0 minutes   **Cooking Time:** 20 minutes

Nutritional Facts: Calories 134, Total Fat 4 g, Carbohydrates 10 g, Protein 8 g

Ingredients

6 cups of brown rice, cooked

1 ½ cups peanut butter, pure

2 cups vegetable broth

2 tbsp canola oil

3-4 cloves of garlic, finely chopped

1 cup green peppers, chopped

1 cup onions, finely chopped

1 cup carrots, chopped, 2 lb firm tofu, cubed

1 cup tomatoes, diced

2 tbsp soy sauce

1 tsp five spices

½ tsp ginger

1 tbsp lemon juice, fresh

Directions

Take a mixing bowl and add in the vegetable stock and peanut butter, then whisk the mixture thoroughly until well combined. Place a large stew pot over medium high heat; add in a little bit of oil and then sauté the onion, carrots, bell pepper and garlic, until the onions are translucent. While this is cooking, season the tofu with the five spices and soy sauce, and then add this in the pot with the vegetables. Cook the tofu until it is browned on all sides, and then pour in the peanut butter mixture, along with the remaining ingredients, except rice. Stir well, bring the mixture to boil, and allow it to cook for 15 minutes on medium low heat. Taste and adjust the seasoning if required, then pour in your serving bowl, serve with cooked rice and enjoy!

Whole Wheat Tortillas

SERVES 12

Prep Time: 19 minutes   **Cooking Time:** 1 minutes

Nutritional Facts: Calories 130, Total Fat 5 g, Carbohydrates 18 g, Protein 3 g

Ingredients

2 cups whole wheat pastry flour

1 tsp baking powder

½ tsp salt

2 tbsp olive oil

½ cup warm water

Directions

Mix the dry ingredients in a bowl after sifting them, to get rid of any lumps, which might be present. Add in the olive oil and stir it until it is well incorporated and a crumbly mixture is obtained. Add a table spoon of warm water one by one, until the mixture starts coming together and then pulls away from the sides of the bowl. Start kneading the dough and keep on kneading until it is soft. Let the dough rest for 10-15 minutes and then when ready take small balls from the dough and using a roiling pin, roll them out into a round flat tortilla. Place a skillet over medium heat, let it heat up and fry each of the prepared tortillas for about half a minute on each side and then place them in a tortilla holder. Cover them with a warm towel to allow them to remain soft and warm. Serve with a salsa and enjoy!

Hoppin John

SERVES 6

Prep Time: 0 minutes   **Cooking Time:** 20 minutes

Nutritional Facts: Calories 145, Total Fat 1.5 g, Carbohydrates 28 g, Protein 4 g

Ingredients

1 tbsp light olive oil

3 cups cooked brown rice

1 cup onions, chopped

¼ cup water

½ tsp basil, dried

2 cups tomatoes, chopped

2 garlic cloves, finely chopped

¼ tsp thyme, dried

1 can of black eyed peas, 16 oz

Pepper and salt, as required

Directions

Place a large skillet over medium heat, drizzle a little bit of olive oil in it and then allow it to heat up. Once the oil is hot enough, add in the onions and cook them until they become translucent. Then add in the garlic and sauté it until the onions start turning golden in color, add the tomatoes, herbs, and cook until the tomatoes have softened. This will take 3-5 minutes.

Then add in the black eyed peas, rice, and adjust the seasoning as required. Allow it to simmer for 12-15 minutes, adding more water of required. Once it is cooked, remove the pot from heat, and pour the pour it into a serving bowl. Serve hot, and enjoy with your friends and family.

Oven Roasted Asparagus

SERVES 4

Prep Time: 5 minutes   **Cooking Time:** 15 minutes

Nutritional Facts: Calories 30, Total Fat 1 g, Carbohydrates 5 g, Protein 3 g

Ingredients

½ tsp Salt

1 lb asparagus, fresh

2 tbsp olive oil

Directions

Trim the asparagus and then drizzle it with a little bit of olive oil. Sprinkle it with salt and make sure that the salt is evenly distributed across the asparagus. Spread the asparagus over a baking sheet lined with parchment paper and then transfer the baking sheet in a preheated oven at 450°F. Let the asparagus bake for 12-15 minutes. Take out, allow them to cool and enjoy. These make for a delectable and healthy snack item.

Crispy Home Fries
SERVES 4

Prep Time: 0 minutes   **Cooking Time:** 20 minutes

Nutritional Facts: Calories 103, Total Fat 3 g, Carbohydrates 11 g, Protein 5 g

Ingredients

4 potatoes, medium, sliced thinly

1 tbsp garlic powder

1 tsp black pepper

1 red bell pepper, chopped

1 tbsp onion salt

1 tbsp oregano

1 tbsp paprika

1 onion, chopped

1 green bell pepper, chopped

1 cup mushrooms, thinly sliced

4 tbsp olive oil

Directions

Place the sliced potatoes in a pot, containing a lid, which fits tightly. Add in the spices and toss them around until thoroughly combined, and the potato slices are evenly coated with the spice mixtures, then set aside.

Take a large frying pan over medium high heat, drizzle a little bit of olive oil, and add in the onions, bell pepper, and mushrooms. Sauté them until the onions are translucent and start getting brown. Add in the spiced potatoes into this mixture and then toss it until evenly incorporated. Once you are done, allow it to sit for 10 minutes over medium low heat. Make sure not to stir the mixture, simply let it sit and allow it to cook. Flip it over and allow it to cook for another 10 minutes. When the chips are golden brown in color from both sides, transfer them to a serving platter, serve and enjoy!

Confetti Pasta
SERVES 4

Prep Time: 5 minutes   **Cooking Time:** 15 minutes

Nutritional Facts: Calories 90, Total Fat 1 g, Carbohydrates 9 g, Protein 6 g

Ingredients

3 tbsp olive oil

2 cups, yellow onions, thinly sliced

½ tsp salt

2 cups cauliflower, chopped

1 cup green beans, trimmed, then coarsely chopped

½ cup parsley, fresh and finely chopped

1 cup snap peas, trimmed and coarsely chopped

1 red bell pepper, diced

6 cloves of garlic, finely chopped

1 lb linguini

2 cups broccoli, chopped

4 green onions, finely chopped

½ cup basil, fresh and finely chopped

Directions

Place the pasta in a large pot filled with water over medium high heat, and then cook it as per the instructions provided on its package. Meanwhile, place a medium skillet over medium high heat and then drizzle a little bit of oil it. Add in the onions, along with the salt and cook the onions until they become soft and translucent, this will take 5 minutes. then add cauliflower and broccoli in it, give it a good stir, and cook the vegetables until they become soft and tender. This would take another 5 minutes. Then add in the bell pepper, garlic, peas, and green beans, and sauté for an additional 5 minutes, taste and adjust the seasoning if required, and then set aside. Place the cooked pasta in a serving bowl, pour the vegetable mixture over it, toss thoroughly, serve and enjoy!

Spicy Spaghetti with Tofu
SERVES 8

Prep Time: 0 minutes   **Cooking Time:** 20 minutes

Nutritional Facts: Calories 79, Total Fat 1 g, Carbohydrates 7 g, Protein 6 g

Ingredients

1 packet 100% whole wheat spaghetti noodles

1/3 cup olive oil

1 ½ packet of tofu, cut into ½-inch cubes\

5 tbsp black olives, chopped

8 oz mushrooms, sliced

3 cloves of garlic, finely chopped

1 ½ tsp chili flakes

½ cup onion, finely chopped

2 cans tomato sauce

1/3 cup basil, finely chopped

Directions

Place the pasta in a cooking pan filled with water, and cook it as per the instructions provided on its packet. Strain and set aside.

Place a non-stick skillet over medium high heat, and then add in a little bit of olive oil in it. Once the oil is hot enough add in the tofu and sauté it, until light brown in color, then remove it from the pan and add in the remaining oil. Place the mushrooms, garlic and onion, into the oil, and sauté it until the onions are soft and translucent. Then add the chili flakes, gives it a stir to thoroughly and evenly combine the spices and then add in the tofu and tomato sauce. Bring the sauce to a simmer and then allow the mixture to cook for 30 minutes or until the tofu is cooked through. Transfer the spaghetti in a serving bowl and then pour the prepared tofu mixture over it, add in the olives and garnish with basil. Enjoy!

Black

SE

Prep Time: 0 minutes

Nutritional Facts: Calories 18, Tot

Ingredients

1 can of black beans, 6 oz, drained and r

1 bunch of cilantro, chopped

½ cup sweet onions, chopped

1 red bell pepper, chopped

1 cup corn kernels, fresh or frozen

The Juice of 5 limes

Salt and pepper, for seasoning

1 mango, peeled and diced

4 warm whole wheat corn tortillas

Directions

Mix all the ingredients together until evenly combined. Leave the mangos, to be added later. Cover with a cling wrap, and place the bowl into a refrigerator and allow it to chill for 20 minutes. Take it out, serve with whole-wheat tortillas and garnish with chopped mangos. Enjoy this healthy and delicious salad with your friends and family.

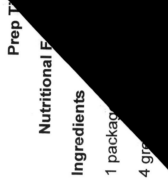

Delicioso Stir Fry
SERVES 4

Time: 5 minutes   **Cooking Time:** 15 minutes

Facts: Calories 45, Total Fat 1 g, Carbohydrates 4 g, Protein 6 g

Dole Cole Slaw

Green onions, sliced

Salt and pepper, for seasoning

1-cup broccoli florets, fresh

1-cup mushrooms, fresh, rinsed and sliced

2 potatoes, peeled, and diced

Olive oil

Directions

Place a large skillet over medium heat, add in 2 tablespoons of olive oil in it and then allow it heat up for 2-3 minutes. Add in the potatoes, and gently toss them in the skillet until cooked but firm from the outside. Remove them from the skillet and then transfer to a plate lined with paper towel, to allow access oil to get absorbed by the towel.

Add another tablespoon of olive oil in the skillet and then pour in the broccoli florets in it. Cook them for 3-4 minutes, until they are cooked, but remain crispy from outside. Transfer to a bowl and set aside. Drizzle a little bit of oil in the skillet and then add in the Cole Slaw and onions, and cook them until the onions start becoming translucent. This will take about 2-3 minutes; make sure to stir it frequently. Add in the mushrooms and toss for another 2 minutes. Once all of the ingredients are cooked, you are ready to serve. Layer the ingredients on a serving plate in the following order; place the Cole Slaw first, followed by the potatoes, and then place the broccoli. Season with salt and pepper and then add the remaining vegetables, serve and enjoy!

Stir Fry Vegetables with Brown Rice
SERVES 4

Prep Time: 1 minute   **Cooking Time:** 19 minutes

Nutritional Facts: Calories 40, Total Fat 1 g, Carbohydrates 4 g, Protein 7 g

Ingredients

3 cups brown rice, cooked

1 tbsp sesame oil

3 green onions, finely chopped

3 tbsp ginger, fresh and finely chopped

½ cup toasted almonds, sliced

¼ lb fresh green beans, chopped

2 carrots, peeled and sliced diagonally

4 cups broccoli, fresh and chopped into bite-sized pieces

2 cloves of garlic, finely chopped

1 can of water chestnuts, finely chopped

2 tbsp soy sauce

4 cups each of kale, spinach, collards, and bok choy, chopped

1 ½ cup peas

Directions

 Place a skillet over medium heat and then add in the oil in it and allow it to heart up for a minute. Then add in the ginger along with the green onions, and sauté for 5 minutes. Once done, add in the green beans, broccoli, garlic, and carrots and allow them to cook for 8-10 minutes. Then add in the kale, spinach, bok choy and collards, toss, and cook for 2 minutes, or until the leaves start wilting. Add in the water chestnuts and stir them thoroughly until evenly incorporated, then add in the brown rise, soy sauce, almonds, and peas. Give it a good stir to combine and then transfer to a serving bowl, serve and enjoy!

Red Lentil Curry
SERVES 4

Prep Time: 2 minute   **Cooking Time:** 18 minutes

Nutritional Facts: Calories 60, Total Fat 1 g, Carbohydrates 7 g, Protein 4.5 g

Ingredients

2 cups red lentils

1 large red onions, diced

1 tsp garlic, finely chopped

1 tbsp vegetable oil

1 tbsp curry powder

1 can of tomato puree, 14.25 oz

1 tbsp ground turmeric

2 tbsp curry paste

1 tsp cumin powder

1 tsp salt

1tsp chili powder

1 tsp ginger root, finely chopped

Directions

Take the lentil and wash them thoroughly with water until the water is clear. Place a pot with water over medium heat, and add the lentils in the water. Cover the pot with a lid and allow the lentils to cook until they are soft and tender, of required, add in more water. Meanwhile, place a large skillet over medium heat, add in the vegetable oil, and place in the onions, to allow them to caramelize. While these two processes are happening simultaneously, take a large mixing bowl, add in the curry paste, chili powder, curry powder, cumin powder, turmeric powder, garlic, salt, and ginger, and mix it together until well combined. Once the onions have caramelized, add in the spice mixture and then cook over high heat for 2 minutes. Make sure to stir continuously, otherwise, the onions might start sticking to the bottom of the skillet and burn. Add in the tomato puree, and reduce the heat to allow the mixture to simmer until the lentils have cooked and are ready to be added into the mixture. drain the lentils and then add then into the curry mixture, stir well to cover the lentils with the curry, transfer to a serving bowl, serve hot and enjoy!

Thai Style Stir Fry with Lemon Grass
SERVES 4

Prep Time: 5 minute   **Cooking Time:** 15 minutes

Nutritional Facts: Calories 40, Total Fat 1 g, Carbohydrates 4 g, Protein 5 g

Ingredients

3 tbsp sesame oil

½ block of tofu, cut into n1/2 inch cubes

2 stems of lemon grass, thinly sliced

1 cup broccoli, chopped

1 red bell pepper, sliced

¾ cup fresh carrots, thinly sliced

1 green pepper, sliced

2 green chilies, minced

¾ cup fresh green beans, sliced

4 cloves of garlic, finely chopped

2 tbsp of lime juice

Salt, for seasoning

Directions

Place a skillet over medium high heat, add in the oil, and allow it to heat up and then add in the tofu. Cook the tofu stirring all the while, until it is golden brown from all sides. Add in the rest of the vegetables and stir for hem for 3-5 minutes, or until they are cooked through and are slightly crunchy from the outside. Add in the rest of the ingredients; cook for another couple of minutes, making sure to toss it thoroughly to ensure that all the ingredients are well incorporated. Transfer to a serving bowl, serve with brown rice and enjoy!

Vegetarian Chili

SERVES 6

Prep Time: 5 minute   **Cooking Time:** 15

Nutritional Facts: Calories 30, Total Fat 1 g, Carbohydrates 5 g

Ingredients

2 green peppers, medium in size, chopped

1 zucchini, sliced

1, yellow onion, medium in size, chopped

1 can of mild green chilies, 4 oz

2 tbsp salad oil

¾ tsp salt

2 cups corn kernels, fresh or frozen

½ tsp red peppers, grinded

1 yellow squash, thinly sliced

2 cans of tomatoes, 16 oz each

1 can of tomato puree, 4 oz

2 cans pinto beans, 16 oz each

2 tbsp chili powder

2 cans black beans, 16 oz each

Directions

Place a large skillet over medium low heat, add in the oil and allow it to heat, and then add in the onions and peppers. Sauté the two vegetables and then add in the zucchini, squashes, corn and red peppers. Cook then until they are soft, yet still hold their firmness, and then add in the green chilies, tomatoes, and beans. Stir them until well combined, and then allow the mixture to come to a boil. Once the mixture has boiled, lower the heat and let kit simmer for 15-20 minutes, stir occasionally. Once cooked, serve and enjoy!

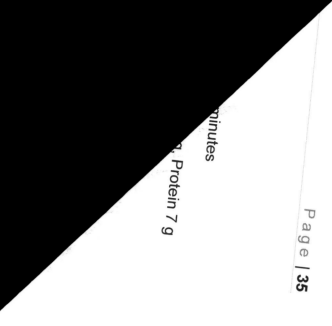

...téed Vegetables

...; 6

...oking Time: 15 minutes

...t 1 g, Carbohydrates 5 g, Protein 5 g

...minutes

...g, Protein 7 g

½ cup carrots, diced

2 cloves of garlic, finely chopped

¼ cup extra virgin olive oil

Directions

Chop and dice the vegetables as instructed in the ingredients. Then drain the white beans, and rinse them with water. Set aside. Place a large skillet over medium high heat, add in the oil, allow it to heat up, and then add all of the previously prepared vegetables. Sauté the vegetables until they are cooked through but still firm and crunchy from the outside. Add in the beans and cook them until thoroughly heated. Give it a stir to ensure that all the ingredients are evenly combined. Transfer to a serving platter, drizzle a little bit of extra virgin olive oil over it, season with salt and pepper, serve and enjoy with your friends and family.

End Note

Daniel Diet is an exciting and impressive way to lead a life which is healthy, without any regrets, and which is in alignment with the biblical way of life. The recipes mentioned in this book are so delicious and yummy that you cannot help but want more. And guess what? They are all healthy, making them an exemplary choice to have during the day.

Try out the recipes given in this book and bring out the culinary talent hidden inside you. Quick and easy to make, they are great to have when you have guests coming over and do not want to burden yourself with too much preparation. When you have a short time at hand, then whip up these recipes in just 20 minutes and amaze your friends and family members with the delectable delights you create through these recipes.

Read the book, go through the recipes, try them out, and feel the exhilaration, which comes with healthy cooking.

Made in the USA
Lexington, KY
24 August 2015